How to Lose Weight Naturally

THE SHORT ANSWER
How to Lose Weight Naturally

PETER WHITWER

Contents

Preface

Special diets, pills, drops, wraps, surgeries—we are obsessed with losing weight. Not with simply losing weight, though, but doing it quickly and easily.

Each new weight-loss fad spurs us to the momentary action, losing a pound or two here and there, but always gaining what was lost—or more—back. A year, a decade, a lifetime of shortcuts leads many to chronic pain, illness, and death.

The short answer to losing weight is much different from the "easy" answer. The main difference is that the short answer provides definite, long-lasting results.

It's time to get healthy.

Step One

Exercise 30 minutes a day.

Exercise Plan

_____

_____

_____

_____

_____

_____

_____

_____

_____

_____

_____

_____

_____

_____

_____

_____

_____

Step Two

Stop eating sugar and processed food, and drink water—at the exclusion of most other drinks.

Healthy Eating Plan

_____

_____

_____

_____

_____

_____

_____

_____

_____

_____

_____

_____

_____

_____

_____

_____

_____

_____

_____

Step Three

Get 7 to 8 hours a sleep
per night.

Sleep Management Plan

_____

_____

_____

_____

_____

_____

_____

_____

_____

_____

_____

_____

_____

_____

Step Four

Be happy.

Happiness Plan

_____

_____

_____

_____

_____

_____

_____

_____

_____

_____

_____

_____

_____

_____

_____

_____